Ginger Alchemy: Transforming Your Health with the Power of Nature.

Preface

Welcome to the enchanting world of "Ginger Alchemy: Transforming Your Health with the Power of Nature." Within these pages, you are about to embark on a transformative journey—one that transcends the boundaries of traditional wisdom and ventures into the realm of modern scientific exploration.

Ginger, with its aromatic allure and rich history steeped in medicinal traditions, emerges as a central figure in this exploration. "Ginger Alchemy" is more than a book; it is an invitation to delve into the extraordinary potential within nature's pharmacy and witness the alchemical magic that occurs when ancient knowledge and modern revelations converge.

The Essence of Ginger

At the heart of this journey lies the essence of ginger—an unassuming root that has adorned the spice racks of kitchens and the shelves of apothecaries for centuries. But "Ginger Alchemy" invites you to see ginger beyond its culinary applications, as we unravel the layers of its bioactive compounds—gingerol, shogaol, zingerone—each contributing to a symphony of healing within the human body.

Bridging Tradition with Science

The pages of this book serve as a bridge between tradition and science. We traverse the ancient landscapes of Ayurveda, Traditional Chinese Medicine, and folk remedies, exploring how ginger has been revered for its therapeutic properties. Simultaneously, we navigate the laboratories of modern science, where rigorous research illuminates the mechanisms that validate the age-old wisdom surrounding ginger.

Culinary Alchemy

Prepare to don the apron and step into the culinary laboratory. "Ginger Alchemy" not only imparts knowledge but also offers a collection of recipes that transform ginger into delectable creations. From savory dishes that celebrate its anti-inflammatory prowess to soothing teas that embrace you in warmth, each recipe is a potion crafted for your well-being.

Ginger in Everyday Life

Witness how ginger seamlessly integrates into the tapestry of everyday life. As you turn the pages, discover its presence in mindful practices, stress management, and even as an aromatic guide in meditation. "Ginger Alchemy" invites you to make ginger not just a spice in your kitchen but a companion in your journey to holistic health.

Personalized Wellness

Recognizing the uniqueness of every individual, this book champions personalized wellness. It guides you in understanding your body's responses to ginger, offering insights into how this remarkable spice can be tailored to your specific needs. Navigate the challenges, consider individual variability, and collaborate with healthcare professionals for a holistic approach to well-being.

The Future Unfolds

As you approach the concluding chapters, gaze into the future of ginger. "Ginger Alchemy" paints a vision where this spice transcends its historical roots, finding new applications in personalized medicine, innovative culinary creations, and synergistic blends with other herbs and compounds. The possibilities are as boundless as the transformative potential of ginger itself.

Your Invitation

Consider this book your personal invitation into the world of "Ginger Alchemy." Whether you are a seasoned wellness enthusiast, a curious explorer, or someone seeking transformative change, these pages hold something for you. Let the alchemical magic of ginger guide you on a journey of discovery, healing, and holistic well-being.

May "Ginger Alchemy" be your trusted companion, inspiring you to unlock the transformative power of nature and embrace the art of living well.

Welcome to the transformative journey—your adventure with ginger begins now.

Akash Gupta

Content:

1. "Roots of Wellness: The Origins and History of Ginger"

2. "Nature's Pharmacy: Unveiling the Healing Compounds in Ginger"

3. "The Spice Cabinet: Incorporating Ginger into Your Daily Life"

4. "Ginger's Journey through Time: An Exploration of Traditional Uses"

5. "Culinary Magic: Cooking with Ginger for Flavour and Health"

6. "Brewing Wellness: Crafting Ginger-Based Drinks for Vitality"

7. "Ginger in the Modern World: From Traditional Medicine to Scientific Validation"

8. "Healing Elixirs: Ginger Recipes for Common Ailments"

9. "Ginger and Beyond: Exploring Complementary Therapies"

10. "Growing Your Own: Cultivating Ginger for a Sustainable Lifestyle"

Chapter 1

Roots of Wellness - The Origins and History of Ginger

Ginger, with its rich history and medicinal roots, has captivated cultures around the world for centuries. In this chapter, we embark on a journey through time to uncover the origins and historical significance of this extraordinary spice, delving into its cultural, culinary, and healing heritage.

Unearthing Ancient Beginnings

The story of ginger begins in Southeast Asia, where the plant's wild ancestor, Zingiber officinale, is believed to have originated. Early human communities in regions like India and China were quick to recognize the aromatic and flavorful properties of ginger, incorporating it into both culinary and medicinal practices.

Ancient civilizations, including the Greeks and Romans, traded ginger along the lucrative spice routes, valuing it not only for its taste but also for its perceived health benefits. As trade routes expanded, so did ginger's influence, making it a coveted commodity across the continents.

Ginger in Traditional Medicine

The historical use of ginger extends beyond its culinary applications. Various cultures, from Ayurveda in India to Traditional Chinese Medicine, embraced ginger for its therapeutic qualities. Its warm and pungent nature led it to be associated with promoting digestive health and alleviating ailments such as nausea and inflammation.

Exploring the ancient medical texts reveals a fascinating tapestry of remedies where ginger was a key player. Whether infused in teas, incorporated into tonics, or applied topically, ginger became a symbol of wellness in diverse healing traditions.

Ginger's Cultural Significance

Beyond its medicinal uses, ginger has played a central role in cultural practices and rituals. In some societies, it was considered a symbol of prosperity and fertility. In others, it was used in religious ceremonies, believed to have purifying qualities that connected the earthly and spiritual realms.

The spice's journey didn't stop in Asia; it traversed the globe, becoming a staple in European and Middle Eastern cuisines. Gingerbread, a beloved European delicacy, became synonymous with holidays and celebrations, showcasing the spice's versatility and cultural adaptability.

The Spice that Sparked Exploration

During the Age of Exploration, ginger became a symbol of wealth and luxury. Explorers like Marco Polo and Vasco da Gama encountered this intriguing spice during their travels, sparking further interest in the far-reaching lands where ginger was cultivated. The spice's allure contributed to the opening of new trade routes, shaping global economies and fostering cultural exchange.

Ginger as a Culinary Delight

Transitioning from its medicinal and symbolic uses, ginger found its way into kitchens worldwide. In this chapter, we explore the spice's role in culinary traditions, from savory dishes to sweets. Ginger's distinctive flavor profile, balancing spiciness and warmth, adds depth to recipes, making it a versatile ingredient in both traditional and contemporary cuisines.

From Asian stir-fries to Caribbean ginger beer, the culinary landscape transformed as ginger became a global culinary ambassador. The chapter delves into specific recipes, historical cookbooks, and the evolution of ginger-infused dishes, showcasing its ability to enhance flavors and create culinary masterpieces.

Ginger Across Continents

As trade routes expanded, ginger became a commodity exchanged between cultures. In this chapter, we trace the spice's journey across continents, exploring how it adapted to diverse climates and cuisines. From the spice markets of Istanbul to the spice gardens of the Caribbean, ginger's global presence is a testament to its resilience and adaptability.

The Evolution of Ginger Farming

Understanding ginger's journey requires examining its cultivation practices. This chapter explores the evolution of ginger farming techniques, from traditional methods to modern, sustainable approaches. The spice's cultivation not only shaped landscapes but also influenced farming communities, contributing to agricultural practices that have endured for generations.

Ginger's Influence on Trade and Commerce

Ginger's impact on trade and commerce is a narrative woven into the fabric of human history. This chapter explores how the spice became a valuable commodity, driving economic exchanges and shaping the destinies of nations. From ancient spice routes to the spice trade monopolies of the 17th century, ginger's economic significance is as compelling as its flavor.

Ginger in Literature and Folklore

Beyond the kitchen and medicine cabinet, ginger has left its mark on literature and folklore. This chapter explores the spice's role in myths, legends, and storytelling traditions. From the tales of the Arabian Nights to folk remedies passed down through generations, ginger's presence in cultural narratives reveals the enduring fascination humans have had with this remarkable spice.

Conclusion

As we conclude our exploration of the roots of wellness, we find that ginger's journey is as much a cultural odyssey as it is a botanical one. From its humble beginnings in the lush landscapes of Southeast Asia to its place on tables and in medicine cabinets worldwide, ginger's history is a testament to the enduring relationship between humans and the natural world. In the following chapters, we will continue to unravel the layers of this captivating spice, exploring its medicinal properties, culinary applications, and its place in contemporary health and wellness.

Chapter 2

Nature's Pharmacy - Unveiling the Healing Compounds in Ginger

Ginger's extraordinary health benefits are rooted in its intricate chemical composition, making it a powerful ally in natural medicine. In this chapter, we delve into the molecular world of ginger, exploring the compounds that contribute to its therapeutic properties and unraveling the science behind its healing potential.

The Chemistry of Ginger

At the heart of ginger's healing prowess lies a complex array of bioactive compounds. Chief among them is gingerol, the pungent compound responsible for the spice's distinctive flavor. Gingerol is a member of the gingerol family, and it is known for its antioxidant and anti-inflammatory properties.

As ginger undergoes various stages of processing or cooking, gingerol transforms into zingerone and shogaol. Each compound contributes uniquely to ginger's therapeutic effects, providing a spectrum of benefits that extend beyond mere taste.

Antioxidant Powerhouse

Ginger boasts robust antioxidant activity, thanks to the presence of gingerol and other related compounds. Antioxidants play a crucial role in neutralizing free radicals — unstable molecules that can damage cells and contribute to chronic diseases. The abundance of antioxidants in ginger positions it as a natural defender against oxidative stress, supporting overall health and longevity.

Anti-Inflammatory Properties

Inflammation is a natural response of the body to injury or infection, but chronic inflammation can lead to various health issues. Ginger's anti-inflammatory properties, attributed to gingerol and other bioactive compounds, have been studied for their potential in alleviating inflammatory conditions such as arthritis and muscle soreness. This chapter explores the scientific evidence behind ginger's anti-inflammatory effects and its implications for holistic health.

Gastrointestinal Comfort

From ancient times, ginger has been revered for its ability to soothe digestive discomfort. This chapter delves into the mechanisms by which ginger promotes gastrointestinal well-being. Whether consumed as a tea, in culinary dishes, or in supplement form, ginger has been associated with easing nausea, reducing indigestion, and supporting overall digestive health.

Cardiovascular Benefits

Emerging research suggests that ginger may contribute to cardiovascular health. This chapter examines the potential of ginger in lowering blood pressure, reducing cholesterol levels, and improving overall heart function. By exploring the interactions between ginger's bioactive compounds and the cardiovascular system, we gain insights into how this spice may play a role in preventing heart-related issues.

Neuroprotective Effects

The relationship between ginger and brain health is an intriguing area of study. This chapter explores the neuroprotective properties of ginger, including its potential in supporting cognitive function and protecting against age-related neurodegenerative diseases. From antioxidant actions to anti-inflammatory effects, the compounds in ginger offer a multifaceted approach to brain health.

Anti-Cancer Properties

Ginger's potential role in cancer prevention and treatment is a topic of ongoing research. This chapter provides an overview of studies investigating ginger's anti-cancer properties. While more research is needed to establish definitive conclusions, early findings suggest that certain compounds in ginger may inhibit the growth of cancer cells and contribute to cancer prevention.

Immune-Boosting Potential

Ginger's reputation as an immune booster is rooted in its bioactive compounds. This chapter explores the ways in which ginger may enhance immune function, helping the body defend itself against infections and illnesses. From its anti-inflammatory effects to its antioxidant activity, ginger's contributions to immune health are part of its holistic approach to well-being.

Pain Relief and Anti-Nociceptive Effects

Traditionally used for pain relief, ginger's anti-nociceptive properties have been a subject of scientific investigation. This chapter explores how ginger may alleviate pain by influencing pain perception and transmission in the nervous system. From menstrual pain to musculoskeletal discomfort, ginger's potential as a natural analgesic is an important aspect of its medicinal profile.

Absorption and Bioavailability

Understanding how the body absorbs and utilizes ginger's bioactive compounds is crucial for unlocking its full potential. This chapter explores factors influencing the absorption of gingerol and related compounds, including culinary preparation methods and the synergistic effects of combining ginger with other foods. By optimizing ginger's bioavailability, we can maximize its health benefits.

Conclusion

As we conclude our exploration of the healing compounds in ginger, it becomes evident that this spice is a true gift from nature. Its molecular complexity, combined with centuries of traditional use and modern scientific scrutiny, positions ginger as a multifaceted remedy for a wide array of health concerns. In the following chapters, we will delve deeper into practical applications of ginger for wellness, exploring culinary delights, medicinal recipes, and lifestyle integrations that harness the full potential of this remarkable spice.

Chapter 3

The Spice Cabinet - Incorporating Ginger into Your Daily Life

Ginger, with its distinctive flavor and multifaceted health benefits, is a versatile spice that can transform ordinary dishes into culinary delights. In this chapter, we explore the diverse ways in which ginger can be incorporated into your daily life, from the kitchen to the medicine cabinet, providing not only a burst of flavor but also a myriad of wellness benefits.

Culinary Artistry with Ginger

1. Ginger in Everyday Cooking:

Ginger's warm and spicy notes make it a culinary treasure. This section delves into the art of using fresh or powdered ginger in everyday cooking, from sautés and stir-fries to soups and stews. Learn how to balance its flavors to enhance both savory and sweet dishes.

2. Baking with Ginger:

The marriage of ginger and baked goods is a timeless affair. Explore the world of ginger-infused treats, from classic gingerbread cookies and cakes to innovative pastries. Discover how ginger adds depth and character to your favorite desserts.

3. Ginger in Beverages:

Elevate your beverage game by incorporating ginger into drinks. From soothing ginger tea to refreshing ginger lemonades and cocktails, this section explores the versatility of ginger in both hot and cold beverages.

Healing Elixirs and Tonics

4. Ginger Tea Remedies:

Uncover the secrets of ginger tea as a remedy for various ailments. This section explores different ginger tea blends designed to address specific health concerns, from digestion and inflammation to cold and flu symptoms.

5. Ginger Tonics for Wellness:

Beyond tea, ginger tonics offer a concentrated form of the spice's healing properties. Learn how to create ginger-based tonics that can be incorporated into your daily routine to promote overall well-being.

Culinary Fusion: East Meets West

6. Asian Inspirations:

Delve into the rich culinary traditions of Asia, where ginger holds a revered place. Explore recipes from Thai, Chinese, Japanese, and Indian cuisines, showcasing how ginger is used to enhance the flavors of diverse dishes.

7. Global Ginger Fusion:

Celebrate the global fusion of flavors by incorporating ginger into non-traditional recipes. From ginger-infused tacos to ginger-spiced pasta, this section encourages experimentation and creativity in the kitchen.

Preserving the Harvest

8. Homemade Ginger Preserves:

Extend the life of fresh ginger by creating homemade ginger preserves. This section provides step-by-step instructions for making ginger jams, pickles, and chutneys, allowing you to enjoy the spice's goodness year-round.

9. Ginger Infusions:

Dive into the world of ginger-infused oils, vinegars, and syrups. These versatile infusions can be used to add depth to a variety of dishes, from salads to desserts, offering a new dimension to your culinary creations.

Ginger in Everyday Health

10. Ginger in Smoothies and Juices:

Discover how to incorporate ginger into your daily smoothies and juices for a health boost. From green ginger smoothies to antioxidant-rich ginger juices, this section explores delicious ways to integrate ginger into your daily wellness routine.

11. Ginger Supplements and Capsules:

For those seeking a convenient option, this section explores the world of ginger supplements. Learn about the different forms of ginger supplements, their potential benefits, and considerations for incorporating them into your health regimen.

Lifestyle Integration

12. Ginger in Skincare:

Beyond the kitchen, ginger offers benefits for the skin. Explore homemade ginger-based skincare recipes, from facial masks to body scrubs, harnessing the spice's anti-inflammatory and antioxidant properties.

13. Aromatherapy with Ginger:

Unwind with the soothing aroma of ginger. This section explores the use of ginger essential oil in aromatherapy, providing relaxation and potentially alleviating stress.

Cultivating Ginger at Home

14. Growing Your Own Ginger:

Experience the joy of cultivating ginger at home. This section provides a guide to growing your own ginger, from selecting the right rhizomes to caring for your ginger plant, enabling you to have a fresh supply at your fingertips.

Conclusion

As we conclude our exploration of incorporating ginger into daily life, the spice emerges not only as a culinary enhancer but as a holistic addition to overall well-being. From tantalizing taste buds in the kitchen to providing remedies in the medicine cabinet, ginger's versatility and health benefits make it a valuable asset. In the following chapters, we will continue our journey into the specifics of ginger's applications, from medicinal recipes to exploring its role in contemporary health and wellness.

Chapter 4

Ginger's Journey through Time - An Exploration of Traditional Uses

Ginger's rich tapestry of traditional uses spans centuries and traverses cultures, making it a spice deeply woven into the fabric of human history. In this chapter, we embark on a captivating journey through time, uncovering the diverse and time-honored ways in which ginger has been utilized for its medicinal, culinary, and cultural significance.

Ancient Roots of Healing

1. Ayurvedic Traditions:

Our exploration begins in ancient India, where Ayurveda, the traditional system of medicine, recognized ginger as a potent healing herb. Known as "vishwabhesaj" or the universal medicine, ginger found its place in Ayurvedic formulations to balance the doshas and treat a myriad of ailments.

2. Traditional Chinese Medicine (TCM):

Crossing over to ancient China, ginger became an integral part of Traditional Chinese Medicine. TCM views ginger as having warming properties, capable of dispelling cold, promoting digestion, and invigorating the body's vital energy, or Qi. Ginger was often prescribed to harmonize the body's internal balance.

Culinary and Medicinal Fusion

3. Medieval Europe:

As trade routes expanded during the medieval period, ginger made its way to Europe, captivating the culinary and medicinal imaginations of the time. In addition to its exotic taste, ginger gained popularity for its perceived ability to ward off the bubonic plague. The spice became a symbol of wealth and was incorporated into both savory and sweet dishes.

4. The Spice Trade:

The spice trade routes of the Middle Ages were the highways through which ginger traveled, connecting East and West. As it journeyed through these trade routes, ginger not only influenced the flavors of various cuisines but also brought with it a reputation for its medicinal virtues.

Ginger as a Culinary Treasure

5. Colonial America:

The colonial era in America marked the introduction of ginger to the New World. Ginger's versatility in cooking and baking quickly earned it a place in colonial kitchens. Gingerbread, in particular, became a beloved treat, with recipes passing from generation to generation.

6. Ginger in the Spice Cabinet:

Explore how ginger became a staple in the spice cabinets of households worldwide. Whether in its fresh, dried, or powdered form, ginger's unique flavor profile adds depth to dishes, enhancing both the savory and sweet dimensions of culinary creations.

Traditional Remedies and Elixirs

7. Ginger in Ancient Remedies:

Throughout history, ginger was a key ingredient in various medicinal concoctions. From teas to tonics, this section uncovers the traditional remedies that featured ginger as a central component, addressing issues from digestive discomfort to respiratory ailments.

8. Herbal Infusions and Tinctures:

Dive into the world of herbal infusions and tinctures, where ginger's medicinal properties are harnessed in concentrated forms. Learn how these traditional preparations were used to address specific health concerns and promote overall well-being.

Ceremonial and Symbolic Uses

9. Ginger in Rituals and Ceremonies:

Beyond its culinary and medicinal roles, ginger found a place in rituals and ceremonies. This section explores how various cultures incorporated ginger into rites of passage, celebrations, and religious ceremonies, where it symbolized purification and good fortune.

10. Symbolism in Folklore:

Delve into the folklore surrounding ginger, where it takes on symbolic meanings in tales and legends. From love charms to protective talismans, ginger's role in folklore reflects the cultural significance attributed to this remarkable spice.

Integration into Modern Culture

11. Revival in the 20th Century:

The 20th century witnessed a revival of interest in traditional remedies and natural healing, leading to a renewed appreciation for ginger. This section explores how the spice regained prominence as people sought alternatives to synthetic medications.

12. Ginger in Contemporary Cuisine:

Trace the evolution of ginger in contemporary culinary landscapes. From celebrity chefs to home cooks, ginger continues to be a star ingredient, adding complexity and depth to dishes that span a wide array of global cuisines.

Preserving Tradition in a Modern World

13. Traditional Practices in a Modern Lifestyle:

In today's fast-paced world, traditional practices involving ginger face challenges. This section explores how individuals and communities strive to preserve and adapt these practices to suit modern lifestyles, ensuring that the legacy of ginger endures.

Conclusion

As we conclude our exploration of ginger's journey through time, it becomes evident that this spice is not merely a flavor enhancer but a symbol of resilience and adaptability. From ancient healing traditions to contemporary kitchens, ginger's versatility and cultural significance have stood the test of time. In the following chapters, we will continue to unravel the layers of ginger's story, exploring its specific applications in health, wellness, and everyday life.

Chapter 5

Culinary Magic - Cooking with Ginger for Flavor and Health

Ginger's journey through the annals of culinary history has been nothing short of magical. Its warm and zesty flavor, coupled with its health-promoting properties, has made it a culinary gem in kitchens around the world. In this chapter, we embark on a flavorful adventure, exploring the art of cooking with ginger to elevate dishes both in taste and nutritional value.

The Versatility of Fresh Ginger

1. Ginger in its Raw Form:

The journey into cooking with ginger begins with the raw root. This section unveils the techniques for peeling, grating, and mincing fresh ginger, showcasing its natural, intense flavor that serves as a foundation for numerous culinary creations.

2. Marinades and Dressings:

Explore the world of ginger-infused marinades and dressings. From Asian-inspired soy-ginger marinades for meats to refreshing ginger vinaigrettes for salads, this section demonstrates how a touch of ginger can transform ordinary dishes into culinary masterpieces.

3. Ginger in Soups and Broths:

Dive into the comforting embrace of ginger-infused soups and broths. Whether it's a classic chicken noodle soup with a hint of ginger or a spicy tom yum soup, learn how ginger enhances the depth of flavors in a bowl.

Sautees, Stir-Fries, and Sautéed Delights

4. Ginger in Stir-Fries:

Stir-fries become a culinary canvas with the addition of ginger. This section explores the techniques of stir-frying with ginger, creating vibrant and aromatic dishes that showcase the spice's ability to marry flavors and textures.

5. Sautéed Vegetables with Ginger:

Elevate the simplicity of sautéed vegetables by introducing ginger into the mix. From ginger-infused broccoli to stir-fried bell peppers, discover how ginger brings a touch of warmth and sophistication to everyday vegetables.

6. Ginger in Sautéed Seafood and Meats:

The marriage of ginger with seafood and meats is a culinary match made in heaven. Learn the art of sautéing shrimp with ginger, or preparing ginger-infused beef stir-fries, unlocking the depth of flavors that ginger imparts to various protein sources.

Baking and Dessert Delights

7. Gingerbread Wonders:

Journey into the world of gingerbread, where the magic of ginger transforms dough into delightful treats. From gingerbread cookies to houses adorned with icing, this section delves into the timeless charm of ginger in the realm of baking.

8. Ginger in Cakes and Pastries:

Explore the sweet side of ginger in cakes and pastries. From moist gingerbread cakes to flaky ginger-infused pastries, learn how to balance the spice's warmth with sweetness for a delectable dessert experience.

9. Ginger-Flavored Ice Creams and Sorbets:

Ginger takes a refreshing turn in frozen delights. Discover how ginger-infused ice creams and sorbets offer a unique and palate-cleansing experience, balancing creaminess with a hint of spice.

Fermented and Pickled Creations

10. Ginger Pickles and Chutneys:

The art of pickling and preserving with ginger adds a zing to meals. This section explores the world of ginger pickles and chutneys, offering a burst of flavor and a crunchy texture that complements a variety of dishes.

11. Ginger in Fermented Foods:

Fermentation becomes a flavorful adventure with the addition of ginger. From ginger-infused kimchi to probiotic-rich ginger kombucha, discover how this spice contributes not only to taste but also to the health-promoting properties of fermented foods.

A Journey through Global Cuisines

12. Ginger in Asian Cuisine:

Asian culinary traditions have long embraced ginger. This section provides a culinary passport, exploring how ginger is used in Chinese stir-fries, Japanese miso soups, Thai curries, and Indian masalas, showcasing its versatility across diverse cuisines.

13. Ginger in Middle Eastern Delicacies:

Middle Eastern cuisine warmly welcomes ginger. Explore the spice's role in dishes like Moroccan tagines, Lebanese stews, and Persian rice dishes, uncovering the subtle yet impactful contribution of ginger to these culinary traditions.

Balancing Flavors with Ginger

14. Ginger in Fusion Cooking:

As culinary boundaries blur, fusion cooking takes center stage. This section explores how ginger acts as a bridge between diverse flavor profiles, creating innovative and delightful fusions that span the globe.

15. Ginger and Spice Pairings:

Understanding the art of pairing ginger with other spices is essential. From cinnamon and cloves to cumin and coriander, this section provides insights into creating harmonious spice blends that enhance the overall taste of a dish.

Conclusion

As we conclude our exploration of culinary magic with ginger, it becomes evident that this spice is not merely an ingredient; it's a culinary alchemist. From savory stir-fries to sweet desserts, ginger's transformative powers in the kitchen are boundless. In the following chapters, we will continue our journey into the medicinal and health aspects of ginger, exploring its role as a healing ingredient in various culinary applications.

Brewing Wellness - Crafting Ginger-Based Drinks for Vitality

In the realm of wellness, few ingredients rival the versatility and vibrancy of ginger. This chapter explores the art of crafting invigorating ginger-based drinks that go beyond mere refreshment, offering a symphony of flavors and health benefits. From traditional teas to contemporary concoctions, join us on a journey into the world of ginger-infused beverages that nurture both body and spirit.

The Elixir of Ginger Tea

1. Classic Ginger Tea:

Our exploration begins with the classic and timeless ginger tea. Dive into the simple elegance of brewing a cup of ginger tea, unlocking not only the spice's robust flavor but also its potential health benefits. From soothing digestive discomfort to providing warmth on a chilly day, ginger tea is a staple in wellness traditions worldwide.

2. Turmeric-Ginger Tea Blend:

The marriage of ginger and turmeric creates a powerhouse of anti-inflammatory and antioxidant properties. Learn how to craft a golden-hued turmeric-ginger tea, not only pleasing to the palate but also promoting overall well-being.

3. Honey-Lemon Ginger Infusion:

Elevate your ginger tea experience with the addition of honey and lemon. This section explores the balance of sweet, tart, and spicy notes in a honey-lemon ginger infusion, creating a comforting elixir that supports the immune system and soothes the throat.

Beyond the Teacup: Ginger Infusions

4. Ginger-Lemon Water:

Simplicity meets hydration in ginger-lemon water. Discover the art of infusing water with the zesty duo of ginger and lemon, creating a refreshing beverage that encourages hydration while providing a burst of flavor.

5. Sparkling Ginger Lemonade:

Beat the heat with the effervescence of sparkling ginger lemonade. This section explores the alchemy of combining ginger syrup with fizzy water, resulting in a thirst-quenching and revitalizing beverage perfect for warm days.

6. Iced Ginger Chai:

Transport yourself to the bustling streets of India with the creation of iced ginger chai. This section delves into the aromatic blend of black tea, spices, and ginger, creating a cooling and spiced beverage perfect for hot afternoons.

Mixology with Ginger

7. Ginger-Mint Mojito:

Ginger takes center stage in mixology with the creation of a ginger-mint mojito. Learn the art of muddling fresh ginger with mint leaves and lime, creating a refreshing and invigorating cocktail that showcases ginger's versatility.

8. Ginger Beer Delights:

Craft your own ginger beer at home, exploring the fermentation process that gives this beverage its effervescence. From classic ginger beer to flavored variations, this section guides you through the steps of creating a zingy and fizzy drink that can stand alone or enhance your favorite cocktails.

9. Ginger Smoothie Creations:

The blending of ginger into smoothies introduces a spicy kick to your morning routine. Explore recipes for ginger-infused green smoothies, tropical fruit blends, and antioxidant-rich concoctions, turning your daily smoothie into a vibrant and healthful experience.

Traditional Elixirs

10. Ginger-Turmeric Shots:

Dive into the wellness trend of ginger-turmeric shots, condensed elixirs designed to provide a concentrated dose of anti-inflammatory and immune-boosting properties. This section explores various recipes and discusses the potential health benefits of incorporating these shots into your routine.

11. Ayurvedic Ginger Tonic:

Ayurveda has long recognized the healing potential of ginger. Discover how to create an Ayurvedic ginger tonic, incorporating other herbs and spices to balance the doshas and promote holistic well-being.

Ginger Mocktails for All Occasions

12. Ginger-Pineapple Mocktail:

Celebrate special occasions with the tropical flair of a ginger-pineapple mocktail. This section provides a step-by-step guide to crafting a non-alcoholic beverage that combines the sweetness of pineapple with the warmth of ginger.

13. Cranberry-Ginger Sparkler:

Toast to festivities with a cranberry-ginger sparkler. This section explores the fusion of tart cranberry juice with the spiciness of ginger, creating a bubbly and vibrant drink perfect for holiday gatherings.

Exploring Global Beverages

14. Ginger Chai Latte:

Embark on a journey into the heart of Indian culture with the creation of a ginger chai latte. This section delves into the preparation of a rich and spiced latte that brings together the comforting flavors of black tea, milk, and ginger.

15. Japanese Ginger Lemon Honey Tea:

Japan's culinary traditions shine in the form of a Japanese ginger lemon honey tea. Learn the delicate art of balancing these flavors, creating a soothing beverage that reflects the grace and precision of Japanese tea culture.

Crafting Herbal Wellness Blends

16. Ginger-Lavender Relaxation Tea:

Unwind and de-stress with a ginger-lavender relaxation tea. This section explores the calming properties of lavender, synergizing with the soothing warmth of ginger to create a herbal infusion perfect for moments of tranquility.

17. Chamomile-Ginger Sleep Elixir:

Create a bedtime ritual with a chamomile-ginger sleep elixir. Discover how the gentle floral notes of chamomile complement the spiciness of ginger, promoting relaxation and restful sleep.

Conclusion

As we conclude our exploration of crafting ginger-based drinks for vitality, it becomes clear that ginger is not only a spice but a tonic for body and soul. From comforting teas to invigorating mocktails, the possibilities are as endless as the spice's health benefits. In the following chapters, we will continue to delve into the medicinal applications of ginger, exploring its role in promoting wellness and addressing specific health concerns.

Chapter 7

Ginger in the Modern World - From Traditional Medicine to Scientific Validation

In the ever-evolving landscape of health and wellness, ginger stands as a timeless remedy that has transitioned seamlessly from ancient traditional practices to the scrutiny of modern scientific inquiry. This chapter unravels the journey of ginger in the contemporary world, exploring how traditional wisdom has merged with rigorous scientific research to validate the therapeutic potential of this extraordinary spice.

Rediscovering Ancient Wisdom

1. Traditional Uses Across Cultures:

The resurgence of interest in traditional medicine has brought ancient practices, including those involving ginger, to the forefront of wellness conversations. This section delves into the varied ways in which different cultures have utilized ginger for centuries, from

Ayurvedic remedies in India to Traditional Chinese Medicine formulations.

2. Ginger in Folk Medicine:

Folk medicine traditions have long revered ginger for its purported health benefits. This section explores the role of ginger in folk remedies, from herbal infusions for digestive issues to topical applications for alleviating pain and inflammation, showcasing the diverse applications rooted in cultural wisdom.

Bridging Tradition with Modern Research

3. Scientific Scrutiny of Ginger:

Modern scientific research has embarked on a journey to dissect the components of ginger, seeking to understand its mechanisms of action and validate traditional claims. This section explores the methodologies employed in scientific studies, ranging from in vitro experiments to clinical trials, highlighting the depth of research dedicated to unraveling ginger's mysteries.

4. Bioactive Compounds in Ginger:

Delve into the biochemistry of ginger, examining its key bioactive compounds such as gingerol, shogaol, and zingerone. This section explores how these compounds contribute to ginger's flavor profile and, more importantly, how they exert potential therapeutic effects on the human body.

Culinary Delights Meets Nutritional Science

5. Culinary Integration for Health:

The fusion of culinary arts with nutritional science has given rise to a deeper understanding of the health benefits derived from ginger-infused dishes. This section explores how incorporating ginger into daily meals not only enhances flavor but also contributes to overall nutritional well-being.

6. Ginger's Role in a Balanced Diet:

Nutritionists and dietitians recognize the role of ginger in promoting a balanced diet. From its anti-inflammatory properties to its potential impact on metabolic health, this section explores how ginger fits into modern dietary recommendations and contributes to holistic wellness.

Digestive Health and Beyond

7. Ginger and Gastrointestinal Well-being:

Scientific studies have shed light on ginger's impact on digestive health. This section examines how ginger may aid in alleviating indigestion, reducing nausea, and supporting overall gastrointestinal well-being, providing evidence-based insights into traditional claims.

8. Anti-Inflammatory Effects:

Inflammation is a common denominator in many chronic diseases. Scientific validation of ginger's anti-inflammatory effects opens new avenues for its potential role in managing conditions such as arthritis and inflammatory bowel diseases. This section explores the research behind ginger's impact on inflammatory pathways.

Cardiovascular Health and Metabolism

9. Cardiometabolic Benefits of Ginger:

Emerging research suggests that ginger may have positive effects on cardiovascular health and metabolism. This section explores how ginger may contribute to lowering blood pressure, improving lipid profiles, and influencing factors related to metabolic syndrome.

10. Ginger and Blood Sugar Regulation:

The relationship between ginger and blood sugar regulation has garnered attention in the realm of diabetes research. This section examines studies exploring ginger's potential role in managing blood glucose levels and insulin sensitivity, offering insights into its implications for individuals with diabetes.

Cognitive Function and Mental Well-being

11. Neuroprotective Properties:

The potential neuroprotective properties of ginger have sparked interest in the scientific community. This section explores how ginger's bioactive compounds may influence cognitive function, protect against neurodegenerative diseases, and contribute to mental well-being.

12. Ginger for Stress and Anxiety:

Traditional practices have often associated ginger with calming effects. Modern research investigates the potential of ginger in managing stress and anxiety, examining its impact on neurotransmitters and stress-related pathways.

Integrating Ginger into Modern Lifestyles

13. Ginger Supplements and Extracts:

The convenience of modern lifestyles has led to the popularity of ginger supplements and extracts. This section explores the different forms of ginger supplements available, discussing their potential benefits and considerations for incorporating them into daily health routines.

14. Functional Foods and Ginger:

The concept of functional foods, those providing health benefits beyond basic nutrition, has given rise to innovative ginger-infused products. From ginger-enhanced beverages to snacks, this section explores how food manufacturers are incorporating ginger into products designed for health-conscious consumers.

Navigating Challenges and Future Directions

15. Challenges in Ginger Research:

Despite the growing body of research, challenges persist in fully understanding ginger's complex interactions with the human body. This section discusses the limitations and hurdles faced in ginger research, encouraging a nuanced approach to interpreting findings.

16. Future Directions in Ginger Studies:

As the field of ginger research evolves, this section explores potential future directions. From exploring novel applications in personalized medicine to investigating the synergistic effects of ginger with other herbs and compounds, the chapter concludes by outlining exciting possibilities for future studies.

Conclusion

As we conclude our exploration of ginger in the modern world, the convergence of traditional wisdom and scientific validation becomes apparent. From the kitchen to the laboratory, ginger's journey reflects a harmonious blend of ancient practices and contemporary research. In the following chapters, we will continue to explore specific health applications of ginger, providing practical insights into incorporating this remarkable spice into our daily lives for enhanced well-being.

Chapter 8

Ginger - A Soothing Balm for Digestive Wellness

In the realm of natural remedies for digestive discomfort, ginger stands as a time-honored champion. This chapter delves into the soothing properties of ginger for digestive wellness, exploring both traditional uses and the scientific evidence that supports its role in alleviating various gastrointestinal issues.

Ancient Wisdom: Ginger's Roots in Digestive Health

1. Ginger in Traditional Digestive Remedies:

The journey into ginger's digestive prowess begins with an exploration of its esteemed place in traditional medicine. Across cultures, ginger has been revered for its ability to ease a range of digestive issues, from indigestion and bloating to nausea and stomach cramps.

2. Ginger Tea for Digestive Comfort:

Among the traditional remedies, ginger tea stands out as a go-to elixir for digestive comfort. This section explores the art of crafting ginger tea, discussing not only its preparation but also its historical use in calming upset stomachs and promoting overall digestive balance.

Scientific Validation: Unveiling Ginger's Mechanisms

3. Anti-Nausea Properties of Ginger:

Modern scientific research has delved into the anti-nausea properties of ginger. From motion sickness to pregnancy-related nausea, studies have shown that ginger may effectively alleviate these symptoms. This section explores the mechanisms behind ginger's anti-nausea effects and its potential application in different scenarios.

4. Ginger and Gastrointestinal Motility:

Digestive wellness is intricately linked to the proper functioning of gastrointestinal motility. Scientific investigations have examined how ginger influences the movement of the digestive tract. This section explores studies that shed light on ginger's impact on enhancing or regulating gastrointestinal motility.

Addressing Indigestion and Bloating

5. Ginger for Indigestion Relief:

Indigestion, characterized by discomfort and bloating after meals, is a common ailment. Explore how ginger may offer relief from indigestion by promoting the emptying of the stomach and reducing symptoms like bloating and discomfort.

6. Reducing Flatulence with Ginger:

Excessive gas and flatulence can be not only uncomfortable but also socially awkward. Scientific studies have investigated the potential of ginger in reducing gas production and alleviating flatulence. This section examines the evidence supporting ginger's role in addressing this common digestive concern.

Inflammation and Digestive Disorders

7. Ginger's Anti-Inflammatory Effects on the Gut:

Inflammation is a common thread in various digestive disorders, including inflammatory bowel diseases (IBD) like Crohn's disease and ulcerative colitis. Scientific research has explored ginger's anti-inflammatory effects on the gut mucosa, offering insights into its potential as a complementary approach in managing inflammatory digestive conditions.

8. Ginger in Irritable Bowel Syndrome (IBS):

Irritable Bowel Syndrome (IBS) is a functional gastrointestinal disorder that affects many individuals. This section delves into studies that investigate ginger's impact on relieving symptoms associated with IBS, such as abdominal pain, bloating, and irregular bowel habits.

Ginger in Gastrointestinal Discomfort

9. Ginger and Gastroesophageal Reflux Disease (GERD):

Gastroesophageal Reflux Disease (GERD) is characterized by chronic acid reflux, leading to heartburn and other symptoms. Discover how ginger may offer relief from GERD symptoms by addressing factors such as lower esophageal sphincter function and gastric emptying.

10. Ginger's Role in Dyspepsia:

Dyspepsia, commonly known as indigestion, encompasses a range of symptoms related to upper abdominal discomfort. This section explores scientific research on ginger's potential to alleviate dyspeptic symptoms, providing insights into its use for overall digestive well-being.

Practical Applications: Incorporating Ginger into Daily Life

11. Ginger in Culinary Creations for Digestive Comfort:

The culinary world offers a delightful avenue for incorporating ginger into dishes that promote digestive comfort. From ginger-infused soups to stir-fries, this section provides practical tips for integrating ginger into everyday meals, enhancing both flavor and digestive benefits.

12. Ginger Supplements for Digestive Support:

For those seeking a more concentrated form of ginger, supplements offer a convenient option. Explore the types of ginger supplements available, their dosage considerations, and potential benefits for digestive health.

Lifestyle Integration for Digestive Harmony

13. Ginger in Traditional Healing Practices:

Beyond consumption, traditional healing practices often involve external applications of ginger for digestive harmony. This section explores the use of ginger compresses and poultices, providing a holistic approach to addressing digestive discomfort.

14. Ginger in Yoga and Mindful Eating:

Digestive wellness extends beyond food choices. This section explores the integration of ginger into mindful eating practices, as well as its symbolic and aromatic role in yoga and meditation for enhancing the mind-gut connection.

Challenges and Considerations

15. Potential Side Effects and Interactions:

While ginger is generally considered safe, it's essential to be aware of potential side effects and interactions, especially in certain medical conditions or when combined with specific medications. This section discusses considerations for individuals incorporating ginger into their digestive wellness routine.

16. Personalized Approaches to Digestive Health:

Digestive wellness is a highly individualized journey. This section encourages readers to adopt personalized approaches, considering factors such as individual tolerance, preferences, and specific digestive concerns when incorporating ginger into their lifestyle.

Conclusion

As we conclude our exploration of ginger as a soothing balm for digestive wellness, the convergence of traditional wisdom and scientific validation becomes evident. From ancient teas to modern supplements, ginger's journey in addressing digestive discomfort is both rich in history and backed by contemporary research. In the following chapters, we will continue to unravel the layers of ginger's therapeutic potential, exploring its applications in addressing various health concerns and promoting overall well-being.

Chapter 9

Ginger's Anti-Inflammatory Effects on the Gut

In the intricate landscape of gastrointestinal health, inflammation can be a disruptive force, contributing to a myriad of digestive disorders. Ginger, with its rich history in traditional medicine, has emerged as a potential ally in the battle against gut inflammation. This chapter delves into the scientific exploration of ginger's anti-inflammatory effects on the gastrointestinal tract, offering insights into its mechanisms and implications for digestive well-being.

Understanding Gut Inflammation

1. The Role of Inflammation in Digestive Disorders:

Inflammation is a complex biological response that plays a pivotal role in the body's defense mechanisms. However, when inflammation becomes chronic, it can contribute to the development and progression of various digestive disorders. This section provides an overview of the role of inflammation in conditions such as inflammatory bowel diseases (IBD), gastritis, and gastroesophageal reflux disease (GERD).

2. Chronic Inflammation and Its Consequences:

Chronic inflammation in the gastrointestinal tract can lead to a cascade of detrimental effects, including tissue damage, impaired gut barrier function, and alterations in the gut microbiota. Understanding the consequences of chronic inflammation is crucial in exploring potential interventions to restore gut health.

Ginger's Bioactive Compounds and Their Role

3. Gingerol: The Potent Anti-Inflammatory Compound:

At the heart of ginger's therapeutic potential lies a group of bioactive compounds, with gingerol taking center stage. This section delves into the properties of gingerol, discussing its antioxidant and anti-inflammatory effects that make it a key player in mitigating inflammation within the gut.

4. Shogaol and Zingerone: Allies in Inflammation Control:

Gingerol is not alone in its anti-inflammatory endeavors. Shogaol, formed through the dehydration of gingerol, and zingerone, derived from the drying process of ginger, also contribute to ginger's anti-inflammatory arsenal. Explore how these compounds complement gingerol in addressing inflammation and promoting gut health.

Scientific Investigations into Ginger's Anti-Inflammatory Action

5. Ginger's Impact on Inflammatory Pathways:

Scientific studies have unraveled the intricate ways in which ginger modulates inflammatory pathways. This section explores the effects of ginger on key mediators of inflammation, such as cytokines and prostaglandins, shedding light on its potential to downregulate these pathways and alleviate inflammation in the gut.

6. Gut Microbiota and Ginger:

The gut microbiota, a complex community of microorganisms residing in the gastrointestinal tract, plays a crucial role in gut health and inflammation.

Scientific investigations have explored how ginger may influence the gut microbiota composition, fostering an environment that promotes anti-inflammatory responses.

Ginger's Role in Inflammatory Bowel Diseases (IBD)

7. Ginger in Crohn's Disease:

Crohn's disease, a type of IBD, involves chronic inflammation of the digestive tract. Studies examining the impact of ginger on Crohn's disease have yielded promising results. This section explores the research that highlights ginger's potential in alleviating symptoms and modulating inflammation in individuals with Crohn's disease.

8. Ginger's Effects on Ulcerative Colitis:

Ulcerative colitis, another form of IBD, is characterized by inflammation and ulcers in the colon and rectum. Scientific investigations into the effects of ginger on ulcerative colitis delve into its potential to mitigate inflammation, reduce oxidative stress, and contribute to symptom management.

Gastroprotective Properties of Ginger

9. Ginger's Impact on Gastritis:

Gastritis, inflammation of the stomach lining, can lead to discomfort and digestive disturbances. This section explores how ginger's anti-inflammatory effects may extend to the stomach, providing potential relief for individuals dealing with gastritis and related symptoms.

10. Ginger's Potential in Gastroesophageal Reflux Disease (GERD):

Gastroesophageal reflux disease (GERD) involves chronic acid reflux, leading to inflammation of the esophagus. Research into ginger's potential impact on GERD examines its ability to modulate acid secretion, enhance lower esophageal sphincter function, and address inflammation, offering insights into its gastroprotective properties.

Integrating Ginger into a Gut-Friendly Lifestyle

11. Culinary Delights for Gut Health:

Beyond supplements, ginger's anti-inflammatory properties can be harnessed through culinary creations. This section explores recipes and culinary tips for incorporating ginger into gut-friendly dishes, offering a delightful and practical approach to embracing its potential benefits.

12. Ginger Supplements for Gastrointestinal Well-being:

For individuals seeking a more concentrated form of ginger, supplements provide a convenient option. This section discusses considerations for choosing ginger supplements, their dosage, and potential benefits for those aiming to support gastrointestinal well-being.

Lifestyle Practices for a Holistic Approach

13. Stress Reduction and Mind-Body Connection:

The interconnectedness of the mind and body is a crucial aspect of digestive health. This section explores the impact of stress on gut inflammation and how mind-body practices, coupled with the inclusion of ginger, contribute to a holistic approach for maintaining gut well-being.

14. Exercise and its Gastroprotective Effects:

Physical activity has been associated with positive effects on gut health. This section discusses the potential gastroprotective effects of exercise and how incorporating ginger into a lifestyle that includes regular physical activity may synergistically contribute to digestive wellness.

Challenges and Considerations

15. Individual Variability in Response to Ginger:

While scientific studies provide valuable insights, individual responses to ginger can vary. Factors such as genetics, pre-existing health conditions, and overall lifestyle play a role in how individuals may respond to ginger's anti-inflammatory effects. This section encourages a nuanced approach to incorporating ginger into a gut-friendly regimen.

16. Consulting Healthcare Professionals:

Before making significant changes to one's diet or lifestyle, it's essential to consult with healthcare professionals, especially for individuals with existing medical conditions or those taking medications. This section emphasizes the importance of informed decisions and collaborative discussions with healthcare providers.

Conclusion

As we conclude our exploration of ginger's anti-inflammatory effects on the gut, the symbiotic relationship between traditional wisdom and modern science becomes evident. From ancient remedies to contemporary research, ginger's journey in addressing gut inflammation is marked by resilience and adaptability. In the upcoming chapters, we will continue to unravel the multifaceted benefits of ginger, exploring its applications in diverse health contexts for comprehensive well-being.

Chapter 10

Ginger and Blood Sugar Regulation

In the pursuit of holistic health, the intricate dance of maintaining stable blood sugar levels is a critical aspect often linked to overall well-being. Ginger, a spice celebrated for its culinary and medicinal attributes, has garnered attention for its potential role in blood sugar regulation. This chapter delves into the scientific investigations and traditional insights surrounding ginger's impact on blood sugar, offering a comprehensive understanding of its potential benefits in supporting metabolic health.

The Complexity of Blood Sugar Regulation

1. The Importance of Balanced Blood Sugar:
Balanced blood sugar levels are essential for various physiological functions. Fluctuations in blood sugar, especially prolonged elevations, can contribute to metabolic imbalances, insulin resistance, and the development of conditions such as type 2 diabetes.

This section explores the significance of maintaining stable blood sugar levels for overall health.

2. Insulin's Role in Blood Sugar Control:

Insulin, a hormone produced by the pancreas, plays a central role in blood sugar control. It facilitates the uptake of glucose into cells, helping to regulate blood sugar levels. Understanding the dynamics of insulin and its interaction with blood sugar is crucial for unraveling the potential impact of ginger on this intricate system.

Ginger's Bioactive Compounds and Metabolic Effects

3. Gingerol and Metabolic Health:

Gingerol, one of ginger's primary bioactive compounds, emerges as a key player in its potential metabolic effects. Scientific investigations have explored how gingerol influences cellular pathways related to glucose uptake, insulin sensitivity, and overall metabolic function, providing insights into ginger's potential role in supporting blood sugar regulation.

4. Antioxidant Properties and Glucose Metabolism:

The antioxidant properties of ginger contribute to its potential benefits in glucose metabolism. This section delves into how ginger's antioxidants may mitigate oxidative stress, a factor linked to insulin resistance and impaired glucose metabolism, thereby influencing blood sugar regulation.

Scientific Studies on Ginger and Blood Sugar

5. Ginger's Impact on Fasting Blood Sugar Levels:

Scientific studies have investigated the effects of ginger on fasting blood sugar levels, providing valuable insights into its potential to modulate glucose homeostasis. This section examines research outcomes and discusses how ginger may influence fasting blood sugar in individuals with varying health statuses.

6. Postprandial Blood Sugar and Ginger Consumption:

The postprandial period, following meals, is crucial in blood sugar regulation. Studies exploring the impact of ginger consumption on postprandial blood sugar levels shed light on its potential to mitigate the after-meal glucose surge, offering implications for individuals aiming to support metabolic health.

Ginger's Role in Insulin Sensitivity

7. Enhancing Insulin Sensitivity with Ginger:

Insulin sensitivity, the body's responsiveness to insulin, is a key factor in blood sugar regulation. Scientific investigations have explored how ginger may enhance insulin sensitivity, potentially reducing the risk of insulin resistance and type 2 diabetes. This section discusses the mechanisms through which ginger may exert its effects on insulin sensitivity.

8. Ginger and Insulin Resistance:

Insulin resistance, a condition where cells become less responsive to insulin, is a precursor to type 2 diabetes. Research into ginger's potential to mitigate insulin resistance offers hope for individuals at risk. This section explores the scientific findings on ginger's effects on insulin resistance and its implications for metabolic health.

Exploring Ginger's Impact on Diabetes Management

9. Ginger in Type 2 Diabetes:

Type 2 diabetes, characterized by elevated blood sugar levels, presents a global health challenge. Studies examining the role of ginger in type 2 diabetes management provide valuable insights into its potential as a complementary approach. This section discusses research outcomes and the considerations for individuals with diabetes incorporating ginger into their lifestyle.

10. Ginger as a Modulator of Glycemic Control:

Glycemic control, the regulation of blood sugar levels, is a primary focus in diabetes management. Scientific investigations have explored how ginger may modulate glycemic control through various mechanisms. This section delves into the research supporting ginger's potential to contribute to comprehensive diabetes care.

Culinary Integration for Blood Sugar Support

11. Ginger in Balanced Diets for Metabolic Health:

Beyond supplements, the integration of ginger into balanced diets holds promise for metabolic health. This section explores culinary tips and recipes that incorporate ginger into meals, offering a practical and enjoyable approach to including this spice in daily nutrition for blood sugar support.

12. Ginger Tea and Blood Sugar Benefits:

Ginger tea, a beloved beverage with a rich tradition, has also been studied for its potential blood sugar benefits. This section explores how ginger tea may contribute to blood sugar regulation and provides insights into its preparation for individuals seeking a comforting and healthful option.

Considerations for Incorporating Ginger into Lifestyles

13. Individual Variability in Response:

Individuals may respond differently to ginger's metabolic effects based on factors such as genetics, existing health conditions, and lifestyle. This section emphasizes the importance of considering individual variability when incorporating ginger into lifestyle choices for blood sugar support.

14. Collaboration with Healthcare Professionals:

Before making significant changes to dietary or lifestyle habits, collaboration with healthcare professionals is essential, particularly for individuals with diabetes or other medical conditions. This section underscores the importance of informed decision-making and the role of healthcare providers in guiding personalized approaches.

Lifestyle Practices for Comprehensive Metabolic Well-being

15. Physical Activity and Ginger's Synergistic Effects:

Physical activity is a cornerstone of metabolic well-being. This section discusses how regular exercise, when combined with ginger consumption, may offer synergistic benefits for blood sugar regulation and overall metabolic health.

16. Stress Management and Its Impact on Blood Sugar:

Stress, a prevalent aspect of modern life, can impact blood sugar levels. This section explores the relationship between stress, blood sugar regulation, and how incorporating ginger into stress management practices may contribute to comprehensive metabolic well-being.

Conclusion

As we conclude our exploration of ginger and blood sugar regulation, the convergence of traditional knowledge and scientific inquiry showcases the multifaceted potential of this remarkable spice. From ancient culinary traditions to modern research, ginger's journey in supporting metabolic health continues to unfold. In the following chapters, we will further unravel the diverse applications of ginger, exploring its role in addressing various health concerns for comprehensive well-being.

www.ingramcontent.com/pod-product-compliance
Lightning Source LLC
Chambersburg PA
CBHW081452250726
48662CB00009B/3051